HackneyandJones.com

Writers and Publishers

HACKNEY & JONES

Want Free Stuff?

HEAD TO:
HACKNEYANDJONES.COM

HackneyandJones.com

How do I feel about myself right now and why?

……………………………………………………………………………
……………………………………………………………………………
……………………………………………………………………………
……………………………………………………………………………

When was the last time I tried something new? How did I feel about it?

……………………………………………………………………………
……………………………………………………………………………
……………………………………………………………………………

When was the last time I cried? How did I feel after?

……………………………………………………………………………
……………………………………………………………………………
……………………………………………………………………………

HackneyandJones.com

Do I sometimes compare myself to others? If so, who and why?

....
....
....
....

What do I think are my best qualities and why?

....
....
....

What elements of my personality do I need to work on and why?

....
....
....
.

HackneyandJones.com

If nobody was watching and nobody could find out, what crazy thing would I love to do and why?

....
....
....
....

What did I want to do as a job when I was younger and why?

....
....
....

How would I like others to see me?

....
....
....

HackneyandJones.com

What was I doing when I felt absolutely on top of the world?

…………………………………………………………………………
…………………………………………………………………………
…………………………………………………………………………
…………………………………………………………………………

Am I surrounded by people who only want the best for me? If so, who? If not, why?

…………………………………………………………………………
…………………………………………………………………………
…………………………………………………………………………

What is my favourite day of the week and why?

…………………………………………………………………………
…………………………………………………………………………
…………………………………………………………………………
.

HackneyandJones.com

When was I at my most sensible? What was I doing and why?

....
....
....
....

Have I ever done something bad and got away with it?

....
....
....

What is my favourite colour and why? How does it make me feel?

....
....
....
.

HackneyandJones.com

What would be the top 5 things on my bucket list and why?

....
....
....
....

How do I deal with anger and why?

....
....
....

What would I love to teach somebody and why?

....
....
....
.

What really gets me excited like a kid and why?

....
....
....
....

Did I have a good childhood? Explain.

....
....
....

Would I be/am I a good boss? Explain.

....
....
....
.

What life lesson hit me hard and why?

....
....
....
....

If I found £250 in cash on the street, what would I REALLY do and why?

....
....
....

Would I forgive a murderer? Explain.

....
....
....

HackneyandJones.com

Do I ever get walked over? Explain.

....
....
....
....

What would I tell my 15-year-old self and why?

....
....
....

Do I believe there is life after death? Explain.

....
....
....

What do I love doing in my spare time and why? How does it make me feel?

………………………………………………………………………
………………………………………………………………………
………………………………………………………………………
………………………………………………………………………

Do I worry about what people think of me? Explain.

………………………………………………………………………
………………………………………………………………………
………………………………………………………………………

Do I like being around animals? How do they make me feel?

………………………………………………………………………
………………………………………………………………………
………………………………………………………………………

HackneyandJones.com

What are my core values in life and why?

....
....
....
....

What can I do at this age that I couldn't do 5 years ago and why? How does this make me feel?

....
....
....

How do I feel when I see somebody cry? What is my immediate unfiltered thought and why?

....
....
....

HackneyandJones.com

Do I believe in therapy? Explain.

....
....
....
....

Do I have an ego sometimes?

....
....
....

Have I ever gossiped about somebody? Explain.

....
....
....

Have I ever broken the law, but got away with it? Explain.

....
....
....
....

When I achieve something, how do I celebrate?

....
....
....

Am I living or existing? Explain.

....
....
....

HackneyandJones.com

What would my perfect day look like?

....
....
....
....

Who is my best friend and why?

....
....
....

How do I feel about being alone?

....
....
....
....
....
....

HackneyandJones.com

When was the last time I lied? Explain.

....
....
....
....

When was the last time I did a good deed? Explain.

....
....
....

How do I feel about being in a crowd?

....
....
....
.
....
....
....

HackneyandJones.com

Who do I want to see again from my school days? Explain.

....
....
....
....

Who do I admire and why?

....
....
....

What am I like when I'm unwell?

....
....
....
....
....
....

HackneyandJones.com

What is something I regret and why?

....
....
....
....

When I'm 90 years old, what do I hope I have done in my life and why?

....
....
....

What would I love to do for the sheer hell of it and why?

....
....
....
....
....
....

Do I prefer reading fiction or non-fiction? Explain.

....
....
....
....

Has somebody hurt me really bad in my past?

....
....
....

If I won the lottery, what are the first 3 things I would do and why?

....
....
....
.
....
....

HackneyandJones.com

Do I enjoy travelling? Explain.

....
....
....
....

What do I feel about sex? Explain.

....
....
....

Have I ever hurt somebody? How do I feel about that now looking back?

....
....
....
....
....

What makes me smile?

………………………………………………………………………
………………………………………………………………………
………………………………………………………………………
………………………………………………………………………

How do I feel about winter? Explain.

………………………………………………………………………
………………………………………………………………………
………………………………………………………………………

If I had to doodle one thing right now, what would it be? Doodle in the space below.

HackneyandJones.com

What was the most expensive thing I ever bought?

....
....
....
....

How do I feel about marriage? Explain.

....
....
....

When I see a couple laughing, what is my immediate thought and why?

....
....
....
....
....

HackneyandJones.com

How do I feel about saying 'I love you' to somebody?

....
....
....
....

When I think of speaking in public, how do I feel?

....
....
....

If I see some litter on the ground, what do I normally do?

....
....
....
.
....
....

If I were born again, what would I do differently and why?

....
....
....
....

What star sign am I?

....
....
....

How do I feel about religion?

....
....
....
....
....

What's my view on politics?

....
....
....
....

What do I immediately think when I see somebody who is homeless?

....
....
....

When was the last time I gave to charity? How did this make me feel?

....
....
....
....
....

HackneyandJones.com

Best book I've read and why?

....
....
....
....

If I wrote a book, what would it be about and why?

....
....
....

When it comes to goals and dreams, what stops me from achieving them and why?

....
....
....
....
....

HackneyandJones.com

Do I enjoy my job? Explain.

....
....
....
....

What do I really think about somebody starting a business?

....
....
....

How do feel about my family? Explain.

....
....
....
....
....

HackneyandJones.com

What do I feel about failure? Explain.

....
....
....
....

What do I immediately think (and do) if somebody criticises me and why?

....
....
....

How would I break bad news to somebody?

....
....
....
....
....

What is my favourite song at the moment?

....
....
....
....

What do I feel about meditation? Have I tried it?

....
....
....

What is a secret nobody knows about me?

....
....
....
....
....

How do I feel when I just lay there listening to my own breath?

....
....
....
....

What makes me different from other people?

....
....
....

What does 'success' look like to me?

....
....
....
....
....

HackneyandJones.com

What trait about somebody else do I wish I had and why?

....
....
....
....

What 3 things (no matter how small) am I grateful for right now?

....
....
....

What is my biggest fear and why?

....
....
....
....
....

HackneyandJones.com

What do I think about the sunrise?

....
....
....
....

Is there life on another planet?

....
....
....

When do I feel at my most vulnerable and why?

....
....
....
....
....

HackneyandJones.com

What does the world need in order to be better than it is right now and why?

....
....
....
....

When was the last time I was wrong? How did it make me feel?

....
....
....

What was my best subject at school and why?

....
....
....
....
....

HackneyandJones.com

How do I feel about sleeping in and why?

....
....
....
....

What 3 things do I need to do in order to achieve a goal?

....
....
....

What job do I keep avoiding and why?

....
....
....
....
....

HackneyandJones.com

Is it OK to be wrong sometimes? Explain.
....
....
....
....

How do I feel about the ocean?
....
....
....

Have I been in love? Explain what happened?
....
....
....
....
....

HackneyandJones.com

Have I ever made an assumption about somebody? Explain.

………………………………………………………………………
………………………………………………………………………
………………………………………………………………………
………………………………………………………………………

What movie can I watch over and over again? Why?

………………………………………………………………………
………………………………………………………………………
………………………………………………………………………

How do I feel about food? Explain.

………………………………………………………………………
………………………………………………………………………
………………………………………………………………………
………………………………………………………………………
………………………………………………………………………

HackneyandJones.com

Have I done anything crazy while being drunk? If so, what? How did I feel after?

....
....
....
....

Where is my favourite place? Why?

....
....
....

What thought goes around my head more than any other? Explain.

....
....
....
....
....

Draw a face of how you are feeling right now in the space below:

HackneyandJones.com

How do I REALLY feel about material things? Explain.

....
....
....
....

Is having a degree important? Explain.

....
....
....

What do I feel about flowers? Explain.

....
....
....
....
....

HackneyandJones.com

Do I think perfection exists? Explain.

....
....
....
....

Have I ever suffered from a mental illness? If so, did I tell anybody about it to get support? Explain.

....
....
....

When I look up in the sky, what do I feel?

....
....
....
....
....

What am I most proud of and why?

....
....
....
....

How do I act in an emergency?

....
....
....

What are my hobbies?

....
....
....
....
....

HackneyandJones.com

How do I handle conflict? Explain.
....
....
....
....

What is my daily routine?
....
....
....
....
....

What do I think and feel when I'm sat at a red traffic light? Explain.
....
....
....
....
....

HackneyandJones.com

When did I feel at my most confident?

....
....
....
....

Do I drink enough water in my day?

....
....
....
....
....

What do I feel about the month of April? Explain.

....
....
....
....
....

HackneyandJones.com

What does freedom look like to me? Explain.

....
....
....
....

Have I ever had to call the emergency services? How do I feel about that situation now?

....
....
....
....
....

Have I denied myself support over something that is playing on my mind? Explain.

....
....

HackneyandJones.com

If I could invite 3 famous people to dinner, who would they be and why?

....
....
....
....

If I could say something now to one of my teachers at school, what would it be and why?

....
....
....
....
....

Do I moan a lot about things? Explain

....
....
....
....

HackneyandJones.com

What is my number one goal for the next 2 months and why?

....

....

....

....

Am I sleeping OK? Explain.

....

....

....

....

....

What are my dreams like?

....

....

....

....

HackneyandJones.com

When I walk out my front door, what's my immediate thought? Explain.

………………………………………………………………………………
………………………………………………………………………………
………………………………………………………………………………
………………………………………………………………………………

When was the last time I saw my doctor?

………………………………………………………………………………
………………………………………………………………………………
………………………………………………………………………………
………………………………………………………………………………
………………………………………………………………………………

In general, do I take care of myself as best as I can?

………………………………………………………………………………
………………………………………………………………………………
………………………………………………………………………………
………………………………………………………………………………

HackneyandJones.com

If I was to write a book, it would be about.......

....
....
....
....

Can I sing?

....
....
....
....
....

What is the greatest challenge each day? Explain.

....
....
....
....

HackneyandJones.com

How do I feel about being in the dark?
....
....
....
....

What do I do with my spare cash?
....
....
....
....
....

Do I like early nights? Explain.
....
....
....
....

Well done!

There were some deep and thought-provoking questions in there.

I bet some of the questions you had never really sat down and thought about.

Moving forward, you are going to commit to three things.

One thing to change, one thing to start and one thing to stop. What are they?

I will change……………………………………………
I will start………………………………………………
I will stop………………………………………………

HackneyandJones.com

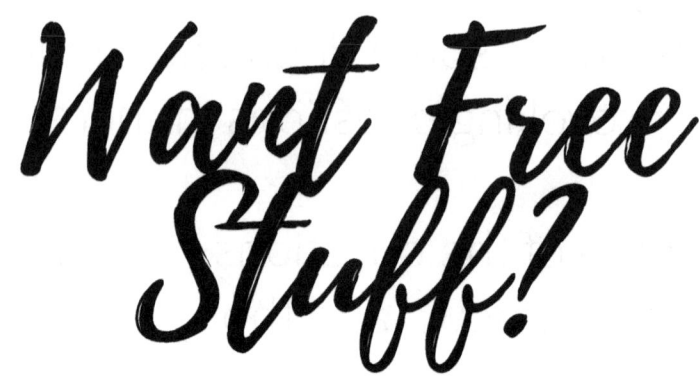

HEAD TO:
HACKNEYANDJONES.COM

HackneyandJones.com

Free Book

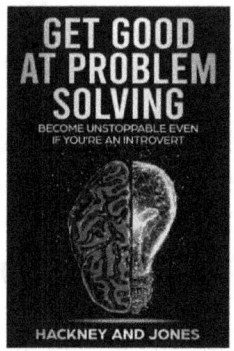

Feedback

IF YOU ENJOYED THIS WORKBOOK AS MUCH AS WE DID IN CREATING IT, PLEASE LEAVE US SOME FEEDBACK ON AMAZON.

WE REALLY DO READ EVERY ONE!

www.ingramcontent.com/pod-product-compliance
Lightning Source LLC
Chambersburg PA
CBHW071126030426
42336CB00013BA/2220